Vegan Fit

10 Vegan Recipes for Pre and Post Workout, To Maximize Energy and Recovery Plus 3 Callisthenic Workouts for Beginners

Table of Contents

Introduction

I want to thank you for choosing this book, 'Vegan Fit - 10 Vegan recipes for pre and post workout, to maximize energy and recovery plus 3 calisthenics workouts for beginners.'

Many vegans think that they are pressed for choice when it comes to pre and post workout meals. However, this is not true, as there are many options to choose from which are capable of providing the body with enough energy and more, both before and after a workout.

Vegan meals consist of fresh fruits, vegetables, grains, pulses, legumes, nuts and seeds and leave out meats and animal derived products such as eggs and dairy. These are capable of providing you with not just energy but also several vital nutrients that are required by your body to remain healthy. However, there is widespread misconception that it is essential to consume lean meats to develop lean muscle. This is absolutely false as it is possible to do so just with the consumption of vegan meals.

If you are on the lookout for simple vegan recipes that can be had as post and pre workout meals, then you have come to the right place! This book will serve as your vegan diet guide and leave you with simple recipes that can enhance your workout routine and help you develop the body of your dreams.

We will also look at three simple calisthenics exercises that you can take up to achieve your weight loss goals.

Chapter 1: Ten Vegan Pre-workout Recipes

1) Death by Chocolate Pudding

Serves: 2

Ingredients:

<u>For the pudding:</u>

- 1 ripe avocado, peeled, pitted, chopped
- ¼ cup cocoa powder, unsweetened
- 2 dates, pitted or 1 tablespoon maple syrup
- 1 medium ripe banana, peeled, sliced
- ¼ cup natural peanut butter
- 1-2 tablespoons dairy free milk

<u>For blueberry cardamom sauce:</u>

- ½ cup blueberries, fresh or frozen
- ½ tablespoon maple syrup
- ½ tablespoon lemon zest
- 1 date, pitted
- ¼ teaspoon ground cinnamon
- A large pinch ground cardamom

Method:

1. To make pudding: Add all the ingredients into a blender and blend until smooth. Taste and adjust the sweetener if desired.
2. Pour into 2 bowls. Cover and refrigerate until use.
3. To make blueberry cardamom sauce: Add all the ingredients of the blueberry cardamom sauce into a blender and blend until smooth. Pour into a bowl. Cover and refrigerate until use.
4. To serve: Drizzle sauce over the pudding and serve.

2) Healthy Peanut Butter Mousse

Serves:

Ingredients:

- 7 ounces extra firm tofu, rinsed, drained, crumbled
- 1 teaspoon vanilla extract
- 1 cup + 6 tablespoons peanut flour
- 14 tablespoons vanilla almond milk, unsweetened
- 1 teaspoon stevia extract
- 1/8 teaspoon salt

Method:

1. To make pudding: Add all the ingredients into a blender and blend until smooth. Taste and adjust the sweetener if desired.
2. Pour into 2 bowls. Serve immediately or cover and refrigerate until use.

3) Mushroom Steel Cut Oatmeal Risotto

Serves: 2

Ingredients:

- 1 tablespoon olive oil
- 1 clove garlic, minced
- 2 tablespoons green bell pepper, minced
- ½ cup steel cut oats
- 2 – 2 ½ cups water
- Salt to taste
- Pepper to taste
- 2 tablespoons onion, minced
- ½ cup mushroom, minced
- ½ teaspoon dried basil
- ¼ teaspoon dried marjoram
- ½ teaspoon dried oregano
- A pinch ground rosemary or 1/8 teaspoon regular rosemary
- 1 tablespoon minced sundried tomatoes
- 1 tablespoon nutritional yeast

Method:

1. Place a heavy bottomed saucepan over medium heat. Add oil. When the oil is heated, add onions and sauté until translucent. Add garlic and sauté until fragrant.
2. Add mushroom, bell pepper and dried herbs. Sauté until the mushrooms are slightly tender.
3. Add oats and sauté for a few minutes until toasted lightly. Add sundried tomatoes and 1-cup water.
4. Lower heat and simmer. Stir frequently to prevent the bottom from burning.
5. When the liquid has dried up, add 1 more cup of water. Stir and simmer until the liquid dries up.
6. Add more water if required and cook until the oats are tender.
7. Remove from heat. Add nutritional yeast, salt and pepper. Stir well and cover for 2-3 minutes.
8. Serve.

4) Tofu Scramble

Serves: 1

Ingredients:

- 1 teaspoon olive oil
- ½ cup red and green bell pepper, chopped
- 7 ounces tofu, rinsed, crumbled
- 1 small onion, chopped
- ½ cup spinach, chopped
- Salt to taste
- Pepper to taste
- Seasoning of your choice to taste (optional)

Method:

1. Place a skillet over medium heat. Add oil. When the oil is heated, add onions and bell pepper and sauté until translucent. Add garlic and sauté until fragrant.
2. Add spinach, salt, pepper and seasoning if you are using. Sauté until the spinach wilts.
3. Serve hot.

5) Breakfast Parfait with Oats and Blueberry Pudding

Serves: 2

Ingredients:

- ¼ cup chia seeds
- 1 teaspoon ground cinnamon
- 1-2 cups blueberries
- 1 small banana, sliced to garnish
- 3-4 cups milk
- 2 teaspoons vanilla extract
- 1 cup old fashioned oats

Method:

1. Add chia seeds, vanilla, almond milk and ground cinnamon into a bowl. Mix well.
2. Add blueberries and stir.
3. Cover and refrigerate overnight. Add more milk if you find it too thick and stir.
4. To make parfait: Take 2 parfait glasses. Make 2-3 layers in the glass alternating with chia pudding and oats.
5. Finally top with banana slices and serve.

6) Stacked Portabella

Serves: 4

Ingredients:

- 4 large Portabella mushroom caps, cleaned, rinsed, pat dried
- 1 cup tempeh, crumbled
- 1 onion, diced
- 2 tomatoes, sliced
- 2 tablespoons olive oil
- 1 tablespoon paprika
- 1 cup cooked quinoa
- 2 cups spinach
- ¼ cup almond cheese, shredded
- 1 tablespoon garlic powder
- 1 tablespoon ground cumin
- 1 tablespoon onion powder
- Sea salt to taste
- Pepper powder to taste

Method:

1. Place a skillet over medium heat. Add oil. When the oil is heated, add onions and sauté until translucent.
2. Add tempeh and sauté for 3-4 minutes. Add quinoa, salt and spices. Mix well.
3. Place portabella mushrooms over a lined baking sheet. Brush the mushrooms with olive oil.
4. Place some spinach over each of the mushrooms. Spread some of the quinoa mixture over the spinach. Stack the tomato slices over the quinoa and finally stack the cheese on top.
5. Broil in a preheated oven for about 5 minutes.
6. Serve immediately.

7) Seitan Stir Fry

Serves: 4

Ingredients:

- 2 tablespoons extra virgin olive oil
- 2 containers White Wave seitan, chopped into bite size pieces
- 1 large green bell pepper, diced
- 1 large orange bell pepper, diced
- Salt to taste
- Pepper to taste
- 4 cups cooked quinoa
- 6 cloves garlic, minced
- Paprika to taste
- 2 avocadoes, peeled, pitted, cut into thin slices

Method:

1. Place a large skillet over medium high heat. Add oil. When the oil is heated, add garlic and sauté until golden brown.
2. Add bell peppers and sauté for 4-5 minutes. Add seitan, paprika and pepper. Sauté for 2-3 minutes.
3. Lower heat and cook for 6-7 minutes. Turn off the heat.
4. Take 4 serving bowls. Add a cup of quinoa in each bowl. Place seitan over it. Top with avocado slices and serve.

8) Protein Power Goddess Bowl

Serves: 3

Ingredients:

- ½ cup green lentils, uncooked
- 1 teaspoon olive oil
- 2 cloves garlic, minced
- 1 medium tomato, chopped
- ¼ cup parsley, minced
- Salt to taste
- Pepper to taste
- ½ cup wheat berries, uncooked or brown rice
- ¾ cup red onion, chopped
- 1 small red bell pepper, chopped
- 2 cups spinach or kale, discard hard stem and ribs, chopped
- ½ teaspoon lemon zest, grated
- Lemon wedges to garnish

For tahini lemon dressing:

- 2 tablespoons tahini
- ¼ cup fresh lemon juice
- 2 tablespoons extra virgin olive oil or to taste
- 1-2 tablespoons water
- 1 clove garlic, minced
- 2 tablespoons nutritional yeast
- Kosher salt to taste
- Freshly ground pepper to taste

Method:

1. To make tahini lemon dressing: Add all the ingredients of the dressing into the blender and blend until smooth.
2. Transfer into a bowl. Cover and set aside for a while for the flavors to set in.
3. Cook the lentils and wheat berries or brown rice according to the instructions on the package.
4. Place a skillet over medium heat. Add oil. When the oil is heated, add onions and garlic and sauté until golden brown.
5. Add bell pepper and tomato and cook until tender. Add spinach and cook until it wilts.
6. Add the dressing, cooked lentils and wheat berries and stir. Lower heat and simmer for 5 minutes. Stir frequently.

7. Turn off the heat and add parsley, salt and pepper. Mix well.
8. Serve in bowls garnished with lemon zest and lemon wedges.

9) Pink Powerhouse Smoothie

Serves: 1

Ingredients:

- 1 cup almond milk or soy milk or cashew milk or hemp milk
- ½ cup cherries, pitted, frozen
- ½ cup strawberries, chopped, frozen
- 1 banana, peeled, sliced, frozen
- 1 scoop plant based protein powder
- 1 tablespoon raw mesquite powder or cocoa powder
- ½ teaspoon pure vanilla extract

Method:

1. Add the milk you are using, cherries, strawberries, banana, protein powder, mesquite powder and vanilla extract into a blender.
2. Blend for 30-40 seconds or until smooth.
3. Pour into a tall glass and serve right away.

10) Super Energy Booster Smoothie

Serves: 2

Ingredients:

- 2 tablespoons raw cacao powder
- 2 tablespoons lucuma powder (optional)
- 2 tablespoons raw maca powder
- 2 tablespoons hemp seeds
- 2 tablespoons chia seeds
- 2 cups almond milk or soy milk or cashew milk or hemp milk
- 1 cup coconut milk
- ½ teaspoon ground cinnamon

Method:

1. Add cacao powder, lucuma powder, maca powder, hemp seeds, chia seeds, milk you are using, coconut milk and ground cinnamon into a blender.
2. Blend for 30-40 seconds or until smooth.
3. Pour into a tall glass and serve with crushed ice, right away.

Chapter 2: Vegan Post Workout Recipes

1) Black and White Bean Quinoa Salad

Serves: 2

Ingredients:

<u>For the salad:</u>

- 3 tablespoons quinoa
- 9.5 ounces canned navy beans, drained, rinsed
- 9.5 ounces canned black beans, drained, rinsed
- 1 small red onion, chopped
- 1 small cucumber, chopped
- 2 tablespoons fresh cilantro, chopped
- 1 small jalapeño, deseeded, chopped (optional)

<u>For the dressing:</u>

- 2 tablespoons extra virgin olive oil or olive oil
- ½ tablespoon apple cider vinegar
- ¼ teaspoon chili powder
- ¼ teaspoon dried oregano
- Pepper to taste
- Salt to taste
- ½ teaspoon ground coriander
- 1 small clove garlic, minced
- 1 tablespoon lime juice

Method:

1. To make dressing: Add all the ingredients of the dressing into a bowl. Whisk well. Set aside for a while for the flavors to set in.
2. Cook quinoa in salted water according to the instructions on the package. Set aside.
3. Add salad ingredients into a bowl. Add cooked quinoa and toss well.
4. Pour dressing on top. Toss well and serve.

2) Teriyaki Tofu Burger

Serves: 4

Ingredients:

- 4 portions extra firm tofu (3 ounces each)
- 2 tablespoons sriracha sauce
- 1 small red onion, sliced
- Butter lettuce leaves to top
- 2 tablespoons teriyaki marinade
- ½ teaspoon red chili flakes
- ¼ cup carrot, shredded
- 2 teaspoons vegetable oil
- Flat out sandwich wraps to serve

Method:

1. Add teriyaki marinade, sriracha sauce and chili flakes into a bowl. Mix well.
2. Add tofu and let it marinate in the mixture for a while.
3. Preheat a grill and place the tofu on the grill. Grill for 3-4 minutes per side.
4. Meanwhile, place a skillet over medium heat. Add oil. When the oil is heated, add onions and sauté until golden brown. Remove from heat.
5. Place 4 flat out sandwich wraps on a serving platter. Place tofu on each wrap. Layer with lettuce leaves followed by carrots and onions.
6. Serve immediately.

3) Simple Vegan Omelet

Serves: 2

Ingredients:

For the omelet:

- 1 ½ cups firm, silken tofu, drained, pat dried
- 4 large cloves garlic, minced
- Salt to taste
- Paprika to taste
- Pepper to taste
- 4 tablespoons hummus
- 4 tablespoons nutritional yeast
- 2 teaspoons cornstarch or arrowroot powder
- 1-2 tablespoons olive oil

For the filling:

- ½ cup onion, chopped
- 1 cup mushrooms, sliced
- 1 large tomato, chopped
- 2 cups spinach, chopped
- Salt to taste
- Pepper to taste
- 2 teaspoons olive oil

For topping:

- 2 tablespoons mixed fresh herbs of your choice, chopped
- 4 tablespoons vegan parmesan cheese
- 2-4 tablespoons salsa

Method:

1. For the omelet: Place an ovenproof, medium size skillet over medium heat. Add ½ tablespoon oil. When the oil is heated, add garlic and sauté until light brown. Remove from heat and cool for a couple of minutes.
2. Add all the ingredient of the omelet including garlic into a blender and blend until smooth. Add a little water if required while blending if the mixture is very thick.
3. Transfer into a bowl and set aside.
4. To make filling: Add oil into the skillet. Place the skillet back on medium heat. When the oil is heated, add onions and sauté until

translucent. Add mushroom, tomato, salt and pepper and sauté until tender.

5. Add spinach and cook until it wilts. Transfer into a bowl.
6. Place the skillet back on heat. Add 1-tablespoon oil. Swirl the skillet so that it is well coated with the oil.
7. Pour half the omelet batter into the skillet. Spread the batter with a spatula or back of a serving spoon.
8. Take about 2 tablespoons of the filling and spread it all over the omelet.
9. Lower heat and cover with a lid. Cook until the edges begin to dry.
10. Remove from heat and transfer into a preheated oven.
11. Bake at 375 F for 10-15 minutes according to the way you like the omelet to be cooked.
12. Take 1-2 tablespoons of the filling and place on one half of the omelet. Let it bake for a couple of minutes. Remove the skillet from the oven.
13. Place the toppings on it. Fold the other side of the omelet over the vegetables and serve.
14. Repeat steps 6 to 13 for the other omelet.

4) Protein Veggie Burger

Serves: 3-4

Ingredients:

- 2 cloves garlic, minced
- 1 small bell pepper, chopped
- 1 small onion, finely chopped
- ½ bunch parsley, chopped
- ½ cup beet, shredded
- ½ cup cooked brown rice
- ½ can black beans
- 1 tablespoon sunflower or nut butter
- ½ tablespoon tamari
- ½ tablespoon ketchup
- ½ tablespoon mustard (dry or sauce)
- Salt to taste
- Pepper to taste
- 1 teaspoon chipotle chili powder
- ½ teaspoon paprika
- ½ cup brown rice flour
- 2 teaspoons vegetable oil
- Cooking spray

Method:

1. Place a skillet over medium heat. Add oil. When the oil is heated, add onion, garlic and bell pepper and sauté until tender.
2. Add the spices, mustard, ketchup and tamari and sauté for a few seconds. Remove from heat.
3. Add beet, brown rice, nut butter and beans into a food processor bowl. Pulse until the mixture is well blended and smooth.
4. Transfer into a bowl. Add the onion mixture and rice flour. Mix well.
5. Divide the mixture into 3 equal portions. Shape into patties.
6. Place a pan over medium heat. Spray some cooking spray on it. Place the patties on it. Cook until the underside is golden brown. Flip sides and cook the other side too.
7. Serve hot with ketchup.

5) Tofu Bento

Serves: 2

Ingredients:

- ½ package extra firm tofu, pressed of excess moisture, pat dried, chopped
- 1 tablespoon low sodium soy sauce
- ½ teaspoon garlic powder
- ½ teaspoon chili paste
- 1 small yellow bell pepper, sliced
- 1 small orange bell pepper sliced
- 1 green onion, sliced (optional)
- 1 small bunch broccolini, chopped
- 1 cup cooked brown rice
- ½ teaspoon ginger, grated
- ½ teaspoon onion powder
- 2 teaspoons olive oil
- Sriracha sauce to taste

Method:

1. Place a skillet over medium heat. Add oil. When the oil is heated, add broccolini and bell peppers. Sauté until slightly tender. Remove from heat.
2. Place another pan over medium heat. Add tofu and sauté until light brown. Remove from heat.
3. To serve: Place ½ cup brown rice on 2 serving plates. Place some tofu over the rice. Top with the sautéed vegetables. Garnish with green onions and serve.

6) Lentil Spinach Soup

Serves: 3-4

Ingredients:

- 1 small onion, chopped
- 2-3 cloves garlic, minced
- 2 carrots, peeled, chopped
- 1 small potato, peeled, chopped
- 3 ounces spinach, rinsed, chopped
- 1 cup dry lentils, green or brown, rinsed
- 2 cups vegetable broth
- 1 teaspoon ground cumin
- Salt to taste
- 7.5 ounces canned or fresh tomatoes, diced
- 1 ½ cups water
- ½ teaspoon smoked paprika
- 1 teaspoon butter or oil

Method:

1. Place a saucepan or soup pot over medium heat. Add oil. When the oil is heated, add onion and carrot and sauté until the onions are translucent.
2. Add garlic, paprika, cumin and salt and sauté for a few seconds until fragrant.
3. Add water, lentils, broth and tomatoes and bring to the boil.
4. Lower heat and cover with a lid. Simmer until the lentils are tender. Add more water or broth if required.
5. Add spinach and cook until spinach wilts. Add salt and simmer for a couple of minutes.
6. Ladle into soup bowls and serve.

7) Chickpea Sunflower Sandwich

Serves: 5-6

Ingredients:

For the filling:

- 2 cans (15 ounce each) chickpeas, rinsed, drained
- 6 tablespoons vegan mayonnaise or tahini
- 2 tablespoons maple syrup or agave nectar
- ¼ cup fresh dill, finely chopped
- 8 pieces rustic bread, lightly toasted
- ½ cup unsalted sunflower seeds, roasted
- 1 teaspoon Dijon mustard or spicy mustard
- ½ cup red onion, chopped
- Salt to taste
- Pepper to taste

For toppings (optional): Use any

- Avocado slices
- 1 large tomato, sliced
- 1 large onion, cut into round slices
- Lettuce leaves, as required

Garlic Herb Sauce:

- ½ cup hummus
- 2 teaspoons dried dill or 2 tablespoons fresh dill, chopped
- Salt to taste
- Water or almond milk, as required
- 2 tablespoons fresh lemon juice
- 4 cloves garlic, minced

Method:

1. To make garlic herb sauce: Add all the ingredients of garlic herb sauce into a bowl. Mix well. Cover and set aside for the flavors to set in.
2. Add chickpeas into a bowl. Mash with a fork. It should not be very smooth in texture.
3. Add rest of the ingredients of the filling except bread and mix well.
4. Place 4 slices of toasted bread on a serving platter. Spread a generous amount of filling over it.
5. Place toppings on it. Drizzle garlic herb sauce. Cover with the remaining 4 slices of bread.

6. Cut into desired shape (optional) and serve with some more garlic herb sauce.
7. Unused filling and garlic herb sauce can be refrigerated for 2-3 days.

8) Black Bean and Sweet Potato Chili

Serves: 2

Ingredients:

- 3 teaspoons extra virgin olive oil
- 1 medium red onion, chopped
- 1 medium sweet potato, peeled, diced
- 2 cloves garlic, minced
- 7.5 ounces canned or cooked black beans, drained, rinsed
- 1 tablespoon chili powder
- ¼ teaspoon ground cumin
- ¼ teaspoon ground chipotle pepper
- Salt to taste
- 7.5 ounces canned diced tomatoes
- 1 teaspoon lime juice
- 1 ¾ cups vegetable stock
- ¼ cup dried quinoa, rinsed

Toppings (optional): Use any

- Avocado slices
- Vegan cream cheese
- Fresh cilantro, chopped

Method:

1. Place a heavy bottomed saucepan over medium high heat. Add oil. When the oil is heated, add sweet potato and onion and sauté until the onion is translucent.
2. Add garlic and sauté for a few seconds until fragrant. Add chipotle pepper, chili powder, salt and cumin and mix well.
3. Add tomatoes, quinoa, stock and black beans and bring to the boil. Mix well.
4. Lower heat and cover with a lid. Simmer until sweet potatoes and quinoa are cooked and the chili is thick in consistency.
5. Add lime juice and salt. Mix well. Remove from heat.
6. Ladle into bowls. Garnish with the toppings and serve.

9) Tempeh Joes

Serves: 2

Ingredients:

- 4 ounces tempeh, sliced into 1 inch thick slices
- ½ tablespoon olive oil + extra for tempeh, if sautéing
- 2 cloves garlic, minced
- ½ can diced or petite-cut tomatoes with jalapeño peppers
- ¼ teaspoon paprika
- 2 whole grain buns
- ½ cup canned chickpeas, rinsed, mashed
- 1 medium onion, chopped
- ½ cup green bell pepper, chopped
- 1 tablespoon chili powder
- 1/8 teaspoon ground cumin

Method:

1. Cook the tempeh by either steaming for 15 minutes or sautéing it in 2 teaspoons olive for 8-10 minutes.
2. When it is cooked, set aside to cool. When cool enough to handle, chop into smaller pieces.
3. Place a skillet over medium heat. Add oil. Once the oil is hot, add onion and garlic and sauté until light brown.
4. Add bell pepper, chickpeas and tempeh. Stir-fry for a few minutes.
5. Add tomatoes, chili powder, cumin and paprika and mix well. Increase heat to high and cook for 2-3 minutes stirring frequently.
6. Split the buns and toast it. Place the tempeh mixture on the bottom half of the buns. Cover with the top half of the buns.
7. Serve immediately.

10) Easy Carrot Slaw with Smoky Maple Tempeh Triangles

Serves: 2

Ingredients:

- 4 ounces tempeh, sliced into triangles
- ¾ tablespoon maple syrup + extra for the slaw
- 1-2 teaspoons tamari or soy sauce
- 2 cups carrots, shredded
- ½ tablespoon curry powder
- Pepper powder to taste
- 2 tablespoons fresh lemon juice
- ¼ cup flat leaf parsley, finely chopped + extra to garnish
- Salt to taste
- Pepper to taste
- 1/8 teaspoon liquid smoke (optional)
- 1 teaspoon extra virgin olive oil or virgin coconut oil
- 2 teaspoons walnuts, crushed
- 2 tablespoons onion, chopped
- 1/8 teaspoon turmeric powder
- 1 tablespoon tahini
- 2 tablespoons raisins (optional)
- Cayenne pepper to taste

Method:

1. Place a skillet over high heat. Add oil. When the oil is heated, add tamari, tempeh, maple syrup and liquid smoke. Mix well.
2. Flip sides a couple of times until brown and the edges darker brown. Remove from heat.
3. Season with pepper and scatter the walnuts over it. Set aside for a while.
4. Meanwhile, add carrots, lemon juice, tahini, parsley, maple syrup, onions, curry powder, turmeric powder, cayenne pepper and raisins into a bowl. Toss well and set aside for a while.
5. Add salt, pepper and lemon juice. Toss well.
6. Divide the slaw into 2 bowls. Place tempeh on top.

Serve right away or chilled

Chapter 3: Calisthenics Exercises

Calisthenics are exercises that you can take up without the need for any equipment. These are ideal for people who do not wish to go to the gym and manage within the confines of their homes.

Here are three simple calisthenics exercises that both men and women can perform.

Crunches

Crunches are some of the easiest and best exercises to carry out at home. They target many different areas of the body and tone the muscles. There are many types of crunches, and some are as follows.

Normal crunch

Regular crunches are those that are performed by a majority of athletes and, bodybuilders to attain a six-pack.

Here is how you can perform them

- Start by lying flat on your back and bend your knees
- Place your feet firmly on the ground and make sure they do not move
- Place your arms at the base of your neck just above your shoulders
- Interlock your fingers and make sure you are in a comfortable position
- Alternatively, you can place your palms behind your head or spread them out
- Now go against gravity to lift yourself up using just your fingers to force you up
- Your legs should remain in the same position and not move
- Try to get up as much as possible before going back down
- It will get easier as you go and you will be able to take your face up to your knees

This exercise tones your abdominal muscles, obliques and also thigh muscles.

Twist crunch

Twist crunches are a variation of regular crunches. They will help you tone your oblique's and laterals.

Here is how you can perform them

- Lie flat on your back and fold your legs
- Place your fingers at the base of your neck above your shoulders

- Lift yourself up and keep your feet glued to the floor
- Once you are in the upright position, twist to the right such that your lower abdomen feels the burn
- Repeat on the left and twist your upper body as much as possible

Bicycle crunch

Bicycle crunches are ideal for all those who wish to put an end to their love handles. It directly affects the muscles that lie in that area and help with toning down the fat. They are also great for toning down lower abs.

Here is how you can perform them

- Lie flat on your back with your legs spread outward
- Place your hands at the base of your neck above your shoulders and interlock your fingers
- Lift your legs into the air so that your thighs are parallel to your stomach
- Now lift your upper torso and twist to the left such that your right elbow touches the left knee
- Go back to the center and twist to the right such that your left elbow touches your right knee
- Keep repeating this until you feel a burn in your lower and upper abdomen
- Try not to take too many breaks in between and keep going at it continuously
- If you feel like you are unable to keep your feet on the ground, then you can get someone to hold your feet in place and perform the crunches. This will make it easier for you to move your upper body

Resistance crunches

Resistance crunches are those where you make use of resistance equipment such as weights to push your body.

Here is how you can perform resistance crunches

- Start off by lying flat on your back and place a weight on your abdomen
- The weight can be a dumbbell or a kettle depending on how much you can take
- Now perform a regular crunch and make sure the weight does not slip off
- You can also perform bicycle crunches if you like

Lunges

Lunges are great for people who wish to work on their legs. They help in toning the muscles and maintaining form. Lunges can be further enhanced by using weights.

Here is how you can perform lunges

- Start by standing upright and place your right leg forward
- Now squat down and try to align your butt with your knee
- Come back to the upright position
- Repeat with left leg
- Make sure you squat as much as you can and repeat the movement as many times as possible without a break
- You can perform walking lunges as that way it will be easier for you to perform many at a stretch
- Lunges can be performed after crunches as they go hand in hand and provide complete body workout

Pull ups/push ups

Pull-ups

Pull-ups target your laterals, biceps and strengthen shoulder muscles. Pull-ups are best if you wish to tone your arms and develop lean, muscular ones.

Here is how you can perform pull-ups

- Start by choosing an area where you would like to perform pull ups
- There has to be a firm rod or surface that you can hold to pull yourself up
- Once you find the area, prepare your body by warming up
- Grip the bar tightly and maintain enough space between your arms to allow your body to come in
- Now put in as much energy as possible and lift your body up
- You must try to touch the rod using your chin
- This might not be possible on the first go and require some degree of perseverance
- As and when you can lift yourself up without too much effort, you can reduce the time taken between pulls
- If you wish to strengthen your biceps and elbows, then grip the bars inwards with your palms facing you. This is known as a chin up
- Alternate between pull ups and chin ups until you feel the burn in your muscles

Push Ups

- Push ups are great to tone your hand muscles as well as chest muscles
- Start by lying face down on the floor and place your palms next to your face
- Now holding them down firmly, push yourself up such that your entire upper body lifts up
- Your toes should be on the floor, and your whole body should be parallel to the floor
- If it is difficult for you to perform this holding your palms to the ground, then you can place your arms on the floor and perform this exercise
- You must lift yourself up and down as frequently as possible to feel the burn

You can do pull-ups and push-ups in repeat sequence as a part of CrossFit training. Do ten push ups followed by ten pull-ups in a minute. Take a small break and repeat.

Conclusion

I thank you once again for choosing this book and hope you had a good time reading it. The main aim of this book was to leave you with pure vegan pre and post workout recipes that you can try out to enhance your routine.

The recipes are simple and make use of fresh ingredients. You need not stick to these alone and can come up with a few recipes of your own. The exercises are all easy to perform and, with regular practice, you can attain the body of your dreams.

I thank you again and hope you have a fun time trying out the recipes and working your way to a healthy, fit body.

Good luck!

9 781974 672899